Through the Years

Jenni Heckendorf

Through the Years

Acknowledgements

David Heckendorf, Ann McMahon, Robin Davidson,
Sarah St Vincent Welch, Emily Beergah, Belconnen Arts Centre

For my mother, Nola Faye Lane

Supported with a grant from the Australia Council
through Belconnen Arts Centre

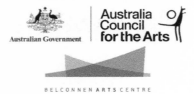

Through the Years
ISBN 978 1 76041 808 3
Copyright © text Jenni Heckendorf 2019
Cover photo: part of Jenni Heckendorf's final assessment
at the ANU School of Art, Canberra.

First published 2019 by
GINNINDERRA PRESS
PO Box 3461 Port Adelaide 5015
www.ginninderrapress.com.au

Contents

1

The Office Window

Sitting at my desk in an inner suburb of Canberra, I try to see my pale pink rose bush through the matted branches of the Japanese maple. Above are fragments of sky, sometimes blue, sometimes white, seldom black and stormy. I stare into one and it becomes a vortex spiralling through the first fifty years of my life, through past events: birth, marriage, deaths and personal triumphs.

To my left are three bookshelves filled with memories; memories of writing courses, the computer-generated art I used to make, and art books, including my favourite artists. I've set aside one shelf for my crystal ornaments and a few old photographs. In front of me is my visual art diploma, old artwork and a calendar. On my right, for most of the time, is my husband, who sits tapping away at his computer.

My typing is quieter. Using my eyes to operate my computer is now my best way of communication. Although it looks difficult for me to look at each letter, it actually eventually will relax me and I can disappear into my own world of writing. Technology is a marvellous thing, especially when you are profoundly physically disabled.

Working with my eyes can become terribly frustrating, especially when my movements are bad. By bad I mean unpredictable, uncontrollable and sometimes even painful. It is worth it. At the end of a long day, I have a chapter of my life on paper. I still need a lot of support. To get this book to publication, I will need extra money for assisted technology and, I imagine then, a person to accompany me in a disability taxi and assist me with communicating with the publisher.

I plan to do as much as I can myself, but it may take less time if I have an extra support worker, as my speech is often slurred.

2

Early Memories

Memories, early memories, are created by stories usually told by family and close friends, with tiny pieces that nudge some unconscious part of the mind.

What I have been told is that I was born to Nola Fay and Kevin John Lane, on the afternoon of 30 September 1958, at Merewether Hospital, Newcastle, in New South Wales. I weighed six pounds and four ounces. Although it was a difficult breech birth, the doctors weren't too worried because everything else checked out as it should. My parents decided that I would be called Jennifer, after a fashion model they read about in the daily paper. I was christened Jennifer Anne at the local church.

My first actual memory is of pulling myself up on the top of a cot rail and squirting chocolate milk over a pale blue wall. Another early memory is of standing on something, putting my short little arm through the wringer of the washing machine. It was a miracle my arm didn't break.

When I was nearly two, we moved to a different house in another part of Newcastle, where the man next door had two peacocks. There was also a sausage dog and a rabbit around the neighbourhood. I had friends my own age, and lots of family.

Family is a confusing thing. When you are young, you think your family is the only way any and every family is. I had a mother, father and sister. I had three cousins. Two of them were girls. My aunties and uncles and Nana and Pop lived in this place called Lismore. I knew it had rock pools and lots of water. It flooded a lot and had sugar cane farms around it. I visited there when I was eighteen months old.

I also had a grandma and grandpa in Newcastle. Grandma had white hair and Grandpa smoked a pipe. They belonged to Dad and he had an auntie and uncle who I later learnt were my great-aunt and uncle, but it took years until I could understand what that meant. The aunties and uncles and Nana and Pop lived in Lismore and they stayed the same number, but I kept getting more cousins. The funny thing was my dad's family in Newcastle kept getting more uncles who then married aunties who had children who were like cousins but weren't cousins. That was because they weren't. My father was an only child, and he called his parents' friends 'Auntie' and 'Uncle'.

In conclusion, for me, all mothers had nanas and pops in faraway places and fathers had family that grew, with a grandma and grandpa and great-aunt and uncle in not so faraway places, and they all had lots of water. Everywhere had lots of water, which made floods and also made the sugar cane grow. Family life was a mum that stayed home and did the housework while children were at school, and a dad that they hardly saw, and aunties and uncles who kept having female cousins and lived far away near the water. Of my eighteen first cousins, seventeen are girls.

One of my 'uncles', Uncle Les, had learnt woodworking in the navy and made me a present for my second birthday; a hand-carved teak canoe. I went to his daughter's first birthday party, where we drank Coke and ate meat pies. Another of these 'uncles', Uncle Jack, would go to Mass with me and Dad. Mum didn't come but she always dressed me up. I wore a brown velvet dress with cream lace and brown ribbon. The organ music overwhelmed me and I burst into tears. Dad used to sing a tune called 'Chantilly Lace' by the Big Bopper, from the year I was born, 1958.

Dad worked at Simpson Pope, a white goods manufacturer. He took me to the warehouse, where there were rows and rows of washing machines covered in dusty plastic. A smell of sawdust filled the whole factory.

3

My New Sister

One day, Mum and Dad took me to a large store where I was to pick out a two-seater bike for myself and the brother or sister who was on the way. I selected a blue and yellow Cyclops.

My sister, Michelle Louise, arrived at about the same time that the right side of my body started having involuntary spasms. My walking became noticeably difficult, my speech was slurred and I shook a little. My right side was dragging along behind my left, slowing me down, making it difficult for me to row my birthday canoe on the Swansea Lake. I couldn't get my chubby little fingers around the oars. I still managed to push Michelle in her pram up and down our front veranda. This is also where I rode what was to be our bike, and played in our blow-up green and yellow plastic swimming pool.

Mum and Dad got me a physio who came to our house. I was allowed to roll around Mum and Dad's bed, doing my exercises. We were only usually allowed to lie in their bed when we were sick. We finished up the exercise session by holding onto the white railing on the front veranda to do balancing and marching exercises. I could see my friend Kim playing across the road.

A year later, I started having convulsions. My 'sleeps', as I named them, could last up to a day. They made me shaky on my feet and I literally needed a hand to get around. I was diagnosed as having epilepsy and probably cerebral palsy.

Cerebral palsy is a condition which can affect all parts of the body or just one limb. There are three main categories with subcategories within them. The main cause of cerebral palsy is lack of oxygen before or during birth. Every fifteen hours, an Australian child is born with cerebral palsy. Research continues and other related causes are being found all the time.

Then my younger sister Michelle was diagnosed with a skin disease, psoriasis. It's funny how children think. I thought every girl with cerebral palsy had a sister with a skin disease.

4

Holidays

I was often sent on 'holiday' while Mum accompanied Michelle to Sydney for treatment for her psoriasis. These holidays included going to my Uncle Henry's farm up near Ballina, where there were stick-like things growing as far as we could see (this was sugar cane). His cows were called Strawberry and Chocolate and his two cats were called Buttons and Bows. If we ate all our vegetables, we were allowed to round up the hens on the big red tractor.

Another time, I stayed in a caravan park. I used my doll's pram to steady myself so that I could still run. There was a tin tugboat, and a bucket and spade that my cousin Kay and I sat and played with in the rock pools.

5

McLeod House

When I was three and a half, my doctor sent me to see another doctor in Sydney, who said I had to stay there for physiotherapy before I could start school. At three years and eight months, I was placed in McLeod House, an institution for children suffering from cerebral palsy who came from the country areas of NSW. Many of the children also had hearing, learning and even sight impairments. I remember a girl from Charlestown was placed at McLeod House at the same time. We both had red boots.

Mum stayed for six weeks to help. Mothers took it in turn to work alongside paid carers doing the day-to-day tasks. It is what they did for their own children at home, but at McLeod House they cared for two or three of us. They dressed us, assisted us with breakfast, then got us ready for school.

From McLeod House we were transported each week day to a school in Mosman. I was lucky enough to have been allowed to go home to our house in North Turramurra. Country children's mothers helped with the day-to-day chores at McLeod House. But when I spent the week at my family home in Sydney, my mother accompanied me to school once a week to help with personal care.

In the afternoon, the mothers greeted us with our afternoon tea, got us ready for dinner, then a bath, and put us to bed. There were no paid staff during the weekdays, so our mums helped with the cleaning and tidying up during the day when we were at school.

One day, I was sick. I remember my mother polishing the floor with a big floor polisher. It vibrated and made a scary whirring sound. The mothers stayed with us until we had our evening bath.

While Mum stayed in Sydney with me, Michelle went up to my grandparents in Lismore. After six weeks, Mum had to go back and look after Michelle. The other kids cried when their parents left, but I didn't. I cried at other times. Staying with different relatives when I was young helped me settle in. I never thought McLeod House was that bad. There were more dolls and other toys to play with than at home. I didn't really miss my sibling. She was only a baby.

After being brought up as a Catholic and having friends attending convents, I looked at McLeod House as some kind of boarding school. After all, we had 'Sisters' and Sunday school, like in Catholic boarding schools, and dumb rules I heard they had. One of ours was not leaving the dinner table until we had all said grace together.

The doctors told my parents I would only be at the Spastic Centre for a year. I would never walk perfectly but they would teach me how to fall and I would be able go to a mainstream school. My 'sleeps' increased, but I saw a trip to the neurologist as a day off school and an electroencephalograph (EEG) as a chance to play with toys. I felt lucky that I wasn't worse off, but then the frequent convulsions damaged my brain further. This meant that I didn't get to attend school in Newcastle with my friends, Alison and Kim. I ended up staying at the Spastic Centre for almost thirty years.

Dad was transferred to Campsie in Sydney, where he was promoted to regional sales representative. This meant I was no longer a country child and I could live at home. Living at home meant an hour's travel each way in an ex-army bus. This bus only went to the Spastic Centre at Mosman. One of the mothers came on the bus with us. The 'city mothers' minded the children on the bus. When we got to school, they helped us out with toileting and lunch preparation. If a child had poor posture, a group of devoted men patiently moulded, padded and covered little chairs which were securely anchored to the bus's floor.

Michelle started seeing a dermatologist in Macquarie Street. My blue and yellow Cyclops tricycle that had driven its way around the yard in Charlestown, now drove up and down the very small balcony of a very small unit overlooking a big football oval.

6

Primary School

Most school mornings we woke up to Dad boiling the jug. He usually had breakfast first and when he kissed us goodbye he got up and went out to the kitchen and had breakfast. After we were dressed and our school bags were packed, I was allowed to watch the morning shows on TV until my bus came. Mum took Michelle to school in the car when I went to school on the bus. Mum came to school with me one day a week. The bus trip took about an hour.

On arriving, we were given our walking frames, crutches, sticks or posture chairs and then the school day would start. No playing in the mornings; they consisted of school lessons interrupted by half-hour therapy sessions. For physiotherapy, we were taken to the ground floor to an enormous room. It had about six little mats for exercising, a parallel bar set up for walking and a plaster room. I was taught to fall forwards and never let my head flop. Many of us had limbs plastered because they were tight and needed to be stretched. This may seem horrendous, but it was just a way of life for us.

All I remember of speech therapy is having ice cubes rubbed over my face to relax the muscles. (I would have thought that it would do the opposite.) There was also an emphasis on suck, blow, chew and swallow. With cerebral palsy, even muscles in the tongue and cheeks can be affected.

It was frustrating to be taught to do everyday things, and when I couldn't quite do them, I felt inferior to my sister and our friends. Trying to feed myself with a fork that had a built-up handle with elastic to hold my hand on wasn't my idea of fun, and the food went everywhere. In the class, we were meant to try and trace numbers that were outlined by small dots. Not being able to control the pencil made me angry.

Then one day in occupational therapy (OT) they taught me to type using a Smith Corona electric typewriter. The typewriter was a strange but complex piece of machinery. Letters were grouped together using different primary colours. The groups of colours were for different fingers, but that didn't really help me. I only ever used my two index fingers on a good day. The guard between the keys did help. I could slide my hands right along it and only press a key if I purposely bent my fingertip. It was best for me to ask the teacher's assistant to put the paper in the roller, so it didn't get crumpled. I could wind in the paper. It made a grinding noise and the keys made a tapping noise. Vowels and consonants were learnt and it wasn't long before I was typing all my schoolwork.

Occupational therapy was fun at first. It concentrated on our hands and arms. We made things and played board games, anything fun that used our hands if we were able. If one of us couldn't use our arms, they would find a part of our body we could use. There is always at least one muscle in the body of a child with cerebral palsy that can be used. (Thirty years later, it could be hooked up to a toy, a game or a computer, for learning.) Fortunately I was pretty good when I was very young. But my shaking got worse every few years. And as my shaking got worse, OT became an escape from schoolwork, which I didn't always like.

After lunch and playtime, it was back to the schoolroom and in kindergarten it was nap time. We lay down on little canvas stretchers. We each had our own cover. I remember getting into trouble for talking to my friend, Wendy, from Newcastle, instead of resting. I also remember the smell of dough. We played with flour and water to make the dough, which was like plasticine.

I despised the straps on the chair that I sat in for hours each day, and undid them whenever I thought nobody was watching, even though I knew they would get done back up. I knew they didn't stop me wriggling and shaking.

A lot of my time was spent in 'recovery'. This was where I had to go when I had a 'sleep'. When I fell out of a billycart, I went to recovery to have the antiseptic gentian violet, or 'purple paint', put on my knees. It was funny to be there without a headache, which was why I usually went to recovery.

A big bell rang for lunch and also at going home time at three-thirty. There was a long corridor leading up to a platform where we got on to our bus. When it wasn't raining, I waited out on the platform with the next load of children for the expected bus, with great anticipation. It would only be an hour or so until I was home with my family.

The day didn't end there. Michelle and I played with friends. We played 'schools' with Susan and Chrissy, our neighbours. We all took on different roles each time we played. If it was my turn to be the teacher, I had to get one of the other girls to write on the blackboard because I was getting too shaky to write. It was taking all my concentration to just stand.

Then there was television. It wasn't so widely used as a childminder back then. The shows we watched were classroom-like, the *Mickey Mouse Club*, *Romper Room* and *Owly's School*. Television was only two years older than me. I literally grew up with Australian television, but television wasn't the pivot of our family. In the backyard we played tea sets with dolls in the tent. We also had a swing. The backyard was our playground.

But the afternoon fun didn't last long. It was taken over by homework, which I did on my typewriter sitting on the floor in the sunroom. Children with cerebral palsy often sat on the floor and crawled around if they were able. This got us out of our posture chairs and enabled us to move around freely.

It was a daily routine for us to have our bath after our homework, but before dinner. Michelle had a 'tar' bath – a bath with strong tar-based antiseptic with a pungent odour. I bathed with her to make her stay in it longer. We drew on the inside of the bath with crayons. If we used all the colours, we could make the water look like mud. Between bath time and our dinner, Michelle had ointments applied to her skin in the lounge room while Mum watched the evening news.

Dinner was meat and three vegetables, Monday to Friday, and we had to sit there until it was all gone, even if it was cold, hard and horrible, or it was no sweets and straight to bed. Dad was often at work during the week, so we just had dinner with Mum in the kitchen. We watched a little bit more television, then went to bed. Mum tucked me in really tight with freshly washed cotton sheets. It felt good because I couldn't wriggle around. I slept on my tummy with an old cloth nappy under my head because I dribbled in my sleep. When the nappies all wore out, I got pretty coloured hand towels to replace them, and they matched the sheets.

If Dad wasn't home by the time Mum put us to bed, I would stay awake until he came home and kissed us goodnight. If he was home, we usually went to sleep to the sound of Mum and Dad chatting about the day, and to the scraping of knives and forks and soft music in the background.

7

Weekends

On the weekends, we played board games: Video Village, Monopoly, Hands Down, Yahtzee and Snap. There were jigsaw puzzles and colouring-in books too. I never managed to keep the colours inside the lines, but somehow I managed to make blobs of colourful scribbles into some kind of picture.

On warm days, we swam in the pool, and visited neighbours, and our cousins, uncles and aunties, Nana and Pop, visited us. We helped weed the garden. We loved the flowers and trees and later our pet dogs, and of course we loved Dad cooking on the barbecue. To this day I love rocks. It must have been our outdoor upbringing that gave me this passion. I still have a rock collection today.

There were chores to be done. While I was still young, thin and flexible, I was able to scamper under and over the bedclothes, straightening the bottom sheet first, then the top sheet, blanket and bedspread. I sat my pillow on top of the side table. I also dressed myself, except for doing up buttons, zips and ties. Sometimes I did the vacuuming, but mainly the edges of the room, and Michelle or Mum would do the middle. My main contribution to the cleaning was dusting the skirting boards. Sometimes if I was fairly relaxed, my job was to iron Dad's handkerchiefs and the back of his work shirts. Some Saturday afternoons we would make cakes, tarts or scones. I could stir the mixture with a wooden spoon, but my movements were too unpredictable to stir scones with a knife.

If Dad wasn't working overseas, we had dinner all together on

Saturday night in the dining room. We weren't allowed to watch TV on Saturday evening if Dad was home, we just talked about our week. When we got the record player, Dad played his music.

Dad had a really nice boss, Mr Gennings. We called him Uncle George, and his wife, Auntie Eadie. When Michelle was really sick in hospital, they minded me while Mum and Dad saw her. They had three really good-looking sons; Robert, John and Bill. We visited their house. It was on the side of a big bushy hill overlooking sparkling water with lots of boats. We drank lemonade and played the board game Hands Down while Dad talked to Uncle George, in their big, posh house.

8

Doctors and Hospitals

My childhood was full of doctors, specialists and hospitals. Doctor Rail was my neurologist. He practised in Macquarie Street in the centre of Sydney. I travelled up to his rooms in an old wooden lift with a door like a cage. Between floors I could see up to the floor above and down to the one below. Doctor Rail's rooms were full of noisy children and anxious parents. The children were bored and the parents were awaiting results.

Before going into Doctor Rail's rooms, I went into a special smaller room for an EEG. It monitored my brain waves. I affectionately called it an egg test. His assistant, an older lady, sat me on her lap and tied a cap-like arrangement on my head. It was made of rubber tubing to form the cap shape, and it was tied under my chin. She rubbed sticky stuff on my head, put clips on the rubber and sang to me. The clips were glued to my head and connected to multicoloured wires which transmitted readings onto paper. Doctor Rail read these papers and was able to tell what was going on in my brain. I called Doctor Rail the Head Doctor because he looked at things going on inside my head.

The Dilantin Doctor Rail put me on swelled my gums and rotted my teeth. Sister Aganor, Sister Wilson and Mum were there when I had an anaesthetic to remove most of my first teeth. It must have been just after Easter because Sister Wilson gave me a pink Donald Duck money box from an Easter Show bag, and put a twenty-cent coin in it. My memory of the rest of the day is a blur.

My arm and facial muscles were affected the most at this stage by the cerebral palsy, but I always thought myself to be luckier than Michelle because I didn't have to have horrible smelly gunk on big red spots. It took me a few years to figure out I should be more than one class above her at school.

From about the age of five or six, I was admitted to Camperdown Children's Hospital nearly every year. It was a brown brick building with a circular driveway that curved around the front of the building, and it also had a circular foyer. The foyer had a lady in a small room with a window in the top half of the door, and a shelf jutting out of it. Mum signed papers for my admission. After that, one of two things happened. The lady, who seemed friendly to me, would escort me to my room, or she called the nurse, who seemed more intimidating, to escort me. It was a different atmosphere up on the wards, the scuffle of nurses running about, sometimes with an urgency, and the clanging of metal instruments and the smell of hospital-grade disinfectant wafted down the corridors. The nurses wore uniforms with white pinstripes on a sky-blue background. They also wore white starched aprons with white origami-like hats.

My first hospitalisation was for a tonsillectomy. I was in a room at the end of a long corridor. There was another cot in there too. I took pride at being in a 'normal'-sized bed. The next thing I remember is waking up with a very sore throat. They gave me ice cream and jelly. To this day, I really dislike ice cream and jelly.

Although the tonsillectomy was the first of many operations I was to have throughout my life, it was the only one that I had at the children's hospital. The other hospitalisations I had there I was poked and prodded by neurologists. Every few years, my shaking and seizures worsened. Neurological teams crowded around my bed, wondering how they could help me next. They usually took me off all my drugs to see what would happen. I believe that I was a guinea pig most of the time.

With treatments came tests: lots of blood tests and EEGs, so that the doctor could see what was happening. The blood tests monitored the levels of drugs in my bloodstream.

My family was always my backup. My mother was a pillar of strength. Mum visited me every day from breakfast to dinner time. If Dad didn't have to work late, he came and visited me in the evenings. Sometimes when Dad visited after work, Mum went home and looked after Michelle, after making sure I did my homework.

I was used to the children's hospital. I regret I wasn't overly interested in the academic side of school, so thought the time in hospital was a kind of school holiday, if a torturous one at times.

9

Home

Meanwhile, we moved to a big old house at Eastwood. Michelle and I had our own large bedroom. My bed had its own cupboard and drawers, but we shared a wardrobe. There was even a separate lounge room with lots of old furniture in it, like Grandma had. It was beautiful, with a pleasant dusty smell.

There was another living room next to the kitchen where we were allowed to play with our toys as long as we cleaned up the mess. Uncle Jack, Dad's friend, who went to Mass with us in Newcastle, often came over and toasted sausages and marshmallows with Dad on a Sunday afternoon. While they were toasting marshmallows, Mum cooked scones to eat with jam and cream in front of the football. Then we watched the Roller Derby. Uncle Jack was a well-built grey-haired man who gave me a blue bird brooch and matching earrings, then promised to marry me when I turned eighteen. Not realising the implications, I felt flattered.

We only spent one Christmas at Eastwood, but I'll never forget it. Uncle Jack gave us a silver Christmas tree. Michelle and I got a swing set between us. One of the swings had a bench seat and the other a horse's head put on back to front, and it had rails around the back and side. I was seven, and asked how come Santa had time to drink a full bottle of beer, eat two pieces of cake and put the swing together back to front? I knew it wasn't Santa. The whole thing didn't make any sense. Some old man couldn't fly through the sky with six reindeer. Only rockets did that, but it would have been wrong to spoil things for

Michelle, so I went along with the story that Santa had lots of helpers. That Christmas I also received a walking frame. It was blue with white handle grips. We also got lots of dolls and Mum and Dad got a new dinner set.

I got one of the first Barbie dolls produced. She was ugly. Her tight, curly chestnut hair reminded me of an old aunt. Michelle had a more modern one. I was jealous of her Barbie, because she had long blonde hair in a ponytail. At the foot of our bed rested a doll's bedroom set – bed, wardrobe, dressing table and chair. We put the dolls in and out of bed, dressed and undressed them, and sat them at the dressing table.

Then there was Easter. I wasn't sure about the Easter Bunny. It didn't make sense but I learnt my lesson after speaking up about Santa. I liked the smell of chocolate in its colourful, shiny foil wrapper. I even liked the rustling noise the foil made when you ripped it off. I usually broke the egg or bunny with my shaking hands but I tried to let the chocolate drop onto the foil.

Easter wasn't such a big deal with our family, except for the Royal Easter Show. We went on rides, got a show bag and a doll on a stick. I liked riding the dodgem cars. When I got my hands on the steering wheel, my arms stopped shaking and I could be in control. I liked putting the balls into the clown's mouth. It was also something I could do on my own without involuntary movements and my hand having to be held. I went to the Easter Show the Tuesday after Easter with my friends in our wheelchairs. They called it a day for the 'Special Children'. To this day, I hate being called 'special'. There are different people. There are people who are sick, disabled people, the elderly and frail, homeless people, and those suffering from things you can't see. Which ones of them are special? It's hard to pick, so nobody is special in my eyes.

Although we only spent a few months at Eastwood, it seems to have been one of the places that made the most impression on me. We took long Saturday drives to Willow Tree Bay, where we hired horses. Dad rented out a light brown pony called Taffy so I could ride it myself. Michelle rode a full-grown horse, but Dad or Mum rode with her most of the time because she was so tiny. Michelle getting the bigger horse and swing made me conscious of being different to other children my age. Being hospitalised helped me understand I wasn't the only one who was different, and certainly didn't have it the worst. My family and friends always let me join in activities with cousins and friends my own age. I often felt dumb when I couldn't do things as fast or accurately as they could, but most of them made exceptions and if they made fun of me, I found a fault in them and made fun back.

Many people called me 'spastic' nastily. To me it just meant I walked funny. Having the Spastic Centre of NSW printed on the side of the school bus didn't worry me until one day a few children my age called me a 'spastic'. It wasn't the word that worried me but the nasty way they said it. I thought for a moment and came to the conclusion it was because my limbs moved when I didn't want them to, and that wasn't so bad anyway. They were the nuts.

Hitting puberty made everything harder. It may have been all those hormones rushing around making me shake more again, but it certainly wasn't an easy transition to womanhood. After many trips to the gynaecologist, it was found I had a double uterus. I had my uterus removed at the tender age of twelve. At the time, all this meant to me was no babies and a lot more swimming. That seemed OK. I didn't know about parents sterilising their disabled children then, so I wasn't angry. At fifteen years old I felt ripped off, but by twenty-five I realised if I couldn't look after my own personal needs, how would I look after those of a baby?

The only thing I was ever shown about sex was a grainy black and white film. It was a bit like an ultrasound. We were only told that the man's sperm were like tadpoles swimming from the penis to the vagina, and nine months later the woman would give birth to a baby. The film never showed how it all happened.

10

Mortality

The same year I started high school, I was back to hospital. This time it was Prince Henry Hospital, the one near Long Bay Gaol. I didn't like this one. I had only ever been to the Children's Hospital at Camperdown and the Women's Hospital in the middle of the city. Prince Henry's wards were big and there were lots of really old people. You couldn't see the other end of the ward. The veranda was closed in, not like the one in Camperdown.

I saw a woman die there. She was next to me. I wanted to talk to her but she wouldn't wake up. I called the nurse over. I kind of knew she was dead, but I didn't want her to be. The nurse shook her saying her name, then pulled the curtain, and it confirmed my suspicions. I'm not scared of dying. I just hope that I fall asleep peacefully and don't suffer like that lady. I am scared of watching people sleep, in case they don't wake up.

By sixteen years, I needed to lie down in the 'recovery' room every day. I started to need longer and longer times to 'recover' each day. Sometimes I needed all day, or I was sent back to McLeod House after lunch. The schoolwork got harder, I got more tired, my level of disability got worse. I became one of the oldest in my class, as others passed me, moving to higher grades.

At the age of seventeen, I spent twenty weeks in Camperdown Children's Hospital, all winter, from 1 May until the 'horses' birthday'. When I wasn't feeling sick, I dictated my work to the teacher at the hospital. Mum read to me. I got my School Certificate and I was delighted.

I went to a neurosurgeon not long after getting my School Certificate and it was decided he would perform brain surgery the following January. I spent the New Year up at Winda Woppa, a small beach town between Newcastle and Foster. 'Uncle' Les's daughters, Lisa and Tracey, came back down to Sydney with us. I had my operation on Australia Day.

I had therapy in hospital after the operation, but I was lucky enough to be able to come home after three weeks. I was allowed to come home early because Mum and Dad could give me hydrotherapy in our own backyard swimming pool.

11

High School

I started high school at the age of fourteen. It was structured differently to primary school. Unlike primary school with grades, high school had forms numbered from one to six. Completing fourth form gave you a School Certificate, and sixth form was the Higher School Certificate.

What really made high school different from primary school for me was the introduction of new school uniforms in the whole school. Children with cerebral palsy can often find it difficult to dress because clothes often don't stretch enough. Some of us couldn't wear the usual cotton school summer uniforms so those who couldn't wore our regular clothes, but with a colour code of green and yellow. It was very patriotic and forward-looking for the time.

Our school badge had a motto, 'Courage and Determination'. I think it is my life motto.

All the classes were held on the ground floor. There was still occupational therapy and physiotherapy, but no school concert, free time, or as many playground activities. Our schoolwork was still done on a typewriter, but now it was marked by correspondence teachers, not pasted in wallpaper-covered exercise books like in primary school, to be marked by class teachers.

We still had class teachers and teachers' aides; but they were more like supervisors. All our work, English, maths, geography and science, was done by correspondence. I was now competing with students from all over the whole country studying through correspondence. Correspondence school was made up mainly of children from the outback and country areas, as well as other marginalised and isolated people. We had individual teachers for each subject, who we never met face-to-face. I took more pride in my high school work than in primary school. I had a different teacher writing comments on my work in each subject and it was motivating. Because this person didn't know my sense of humour, individual habits or quirks, I took more notice of the feedback. Even though we had our separate teachers for separate subjects, the class teacher still played a role, and the teacher's aide helped us with the more physically challenging tasks such as collating and stapling our work that was to be sent away for correction, and then to be returned with comments, and hopefully ticks and not crosses.

Our class had around twelve students. I was the youngest until my disability started increasing. The students in this class ranged in age from about thirteen to nineteen. A thirteen-year-old with a mild disability may be doing the same work as a sixteen-year-old with a severe disability, or vice versa. There are five different categories of cerebral palsy, although different countries use slightly different categorisations. One thing that doesn't differ is that there are definitely different types. And they are not mutually exclusive. Some people have more than one type. And in our class we probably had them all.

My mother had health issues at this time as well. She had three major operations on her stomach. This made it hard for her to walk me about the house. My involuntary movements increased even more. I was advised by doctors to use a wheelchair. This would prevent me from knocking myself about. There were no drugs at that time that could control my movements any more. So I was put back into McLeod House for five days a week.

Being in a wheelchair was a newfound freedom. Instead of taking twenty minutes to crawl down the hallway in our house, I was able to push myself up a corridor almost three times as long in about two minutes. When I reached my destination, I still had the energy to talk to friends and to join in games. I was lucky enough to be able to pull myself up on rails and walk a few yards. Many of my friends could not even do that.

Going home started to become a real chore. Walking was harder there, and there was nothing for me to do without my parents' assistance. I felt like an obligation to them. I loved my family very much and they looked forward to my going home on the weekends, but when I was there I missed my friends and freedom of movement. There was plenty to do there. At McLeod House I was in the Social Club. We had a dance at Mosman every month, which I really enjoyed. They always had a theme. Once, I went dressed up as a Rhoda, my favourite TV star.

12

My Big Operation

When I was eighteen I had major brain surgery. That sounds scary. It was. But it was scarier for those around me. My shaking had got so bad by my late teens I once shook myself out of a hospital bed. All the drugs the doctors tried didn't work. The surgery I had I think was mainly used in Parkinson's patients. There's not much more I can tell you. I think the brain has a coping mechanism, to block out bad things like that. I can't remember the experience in detail.

I do remember that I went on a lovely holiday at Hawks Nest, a beach town on the mid-NSW coast. It was just after Christmas in 1978. Tracey, the daughter of a friend of Dad's , came back to Sydney with us and went home to Newcastle just before the long weekend in January, just before I went to the Royal North Shore Hospital. I vaguely knew what was happening. It was for my brain operation. Sometimes actions speak louder than words. Tracey never came back to Sydney after the summer holidays. I knew something was going to happen and it was something big, but nothing could have prepared me for the experience of how big it was.

After I went through the admission administration, I was taken to a four-person room. My next memory is of lying in the pre-op room. The doctor came in. I asked whether it would be very painful. He said, 'Yes, you will have the worst headache you've had in your life.' Seeing I was used to headaches, as I had one nearly every day, I wasn't too worried.

When I woke up in intensive care, I really did have the worst headache I'd had in my life. Although I had never smashed my head against a brick wall, I thought it felt like that might feel. The nurses had bandaged my ear so it bent over. I did have a really bad headache, but when the nurses asked how I was feeling and I said my ear hurt, they told me, 'You mean your head.' A few days later, when I convinced the nursing staff the operation hadn't affected my sense of where the pain was, they cut the bandages around my ear and found my ear had been bandaged incorrectly and my ear was bruised.

My next memory is of lying down and Mum sitting next to me holding my hand and her saying, 'It's not shaking.' My first exercise was to grip my hairbrush, and the next to grip my toothbrush. When I was able to grip properly, it was off to physiotherapy for me. I can't recall exactly what I did in physio, but I remember at that point it was difficult. I remember being pushed around the nurses' station and being told by the doctor I couldn't go home until I was stronger. I proved him wrong by hitting him in the thigh. I was strong. Mum and Dad assured him they would continue my rehab by making me swim every day. So I finally got out of the hospital. This was a huge life changing experience and I was glad to get back to my family home.

To my disgust, I went back to school for more post-operative intensive physiotherapy to get my left side moving again. So I did a course in commerce also run by the correspondence school. I did not do my Higher School Certificate because I did not want to still be at school when I was nineteen or twenty.

13

'Work'

In November that year, we were all shown a film of Centre Industries, a sheltered workshop run by the Spastic Centre (now the Cerebral Palsy Alliance) which was on the same land as McLeod House, the hostel for children with cerebral palsy. I was led to believe that it was all there was out there for me, employment wise. I did a week of tests and assessments to qualify to work there. By the end of the week, I wasn't sure whether I would have been better off staying at school, if this was what the big wide world was, and my optimism was replaced by a sense of futility.

As my twenty-first birthday approached, I realised I had never thought of getting this old. I was a real adult now, yet I was treated like a child. I was in a teenage dorm and I had people younger than me helping me with my day-to-day needs.

I had a wonderful twenty-first birthday at the Gold Coast with my relatives. I felt I was an adult for a fortnight. Coming back to the same place of work and thinking my only chance of achieving anything was within the grounds of the Spastic Centre was distressing. I was an active member of the Venturers and taught groups of Brownies. I enjoyed talking to the Brownies and the experience showed me I could be a mentor, and I wanted to become a Brownie leader at that time. I gave talks to the Brownies only for a few weeks. Then I became too old to be a Venturer. In my heart, I knew I had to get out of the centre.

I eventually got over my fear of old age and consoled myself that I could have some kind of a future. A few of my girlfriends were moving out to community housing and were given more choice about how they lived. My mother told me that I was too handicapped to move out. I didn't argue, but I joined committees and saw people more handicapped than me moving into the community. I knew she was wrong.

A young man called David joined me working in the sheltered workshop. After only six months of this repetitive job, he complained and was promoted to the office. This was on the top floor. Being on the top floor sounded impressive in itself. There he learnt to program computers. Unfortunately when I went to the office, it was found that the computer card numbers I entered were often written in the wrong order, or backwards. I was said to be 'dyslexic', and it was back to the factory floor for me. As my 'dyslexia' was never treated, I wonder if this was true.

I thought I had been fortunate to have worked upstairs for three months in Computer Services. There wasn't even a view of Allambie Road or anything much to look at. It was the atmosphere. Everybody was so friendly and in that short time I worked quite hard and did earn more money. The reason I made mistakes was because I was not used to looking at the visual display unit all the time. I was used to typewriters.

I then ended up working in the typing pool, which was meant to sound impressive. It was set up in the old craft room (which was quite a large room with old paint stains from its former use, and it was also being used as a dumping ground for old office equipment). In reality it didn't seem so impressive.

By 1985, Centre Industries was abuzz with talk of 'normalisation'. My supervisor told me that normalisation meant being treated at our own individual intellectual age level. That left me confused as to what my intellectual age actually was. We needed to understand this to work on getting a pay rise. I wondered how we could dare ask for a pay rise? We weren't working in a 'normal' working environment. We typed the headings on time sheets and filed and distributed them to 'production teams'. This was where the responsibility ended for most of us. We weren't earning much more money, or even learning simple office skills. I didn't even know what normal intellectual ages were. It was confusing.

14

Falling in Love

David Winston Heckendorf was only seventeen years old when we became friends at McLeod House. David was eight years my junior. When he was in his last year at school, I was doing a bookkeeping course. It was at the beginning of computers. They said nothing would come of me learning bookkeeping because everything was written by hand. They were certainly wrong about that.

David and I met in the homework room. We were meant to be studying. That is when we grew together. I fought it. I thought a seventeen-year-old kid was too young for a twenty-five-year-old woman.

I was attracted to David and would spend hours listening to him philosophising about life in general. Although he made so much sense, listening to him made me feel uncomfortable. I was scared to fall for this kid, yet being with him seemed so right.

As I recall, our first tender moment was on a large carpet in the pool room. I was watching teenage boys playing crab soccer. It is a game of two teams, and the players must keep three limbs on the ground and hit a ball with the other limb. So that night it was boys vs girls. I was the one that asked the girl to not knock out David so the girls' side would win. Suddenly the room emptied; the recreation officer shut the heavy squeaky sliding door and I remember David's large muscly arm cushioned my head, as it does to this day.

15

Committee Work

Throughout these years I also worked on committees. In the early eighties, a group of older people with cerebral palsy set up the 'Office'. The Office was a place we were allowed to express our opinions, discuss our rights, share them, and act as our own advocates. I remember once a colleague of mine was ringing a radio station on a chat line. I forget the subject. He could only talk through a synthesised robotic voice. 'Can you help me?' his voice said. 'Are you for real?' the radio jockey said. My colleague tried to ask his question and got hung up on. We all thought it was funny.

That was one of my first interactions with what went on in 'the outside world'.

The Year of the Disabled, in 1982, brought about a lot of changes for thousands of disabled people. People with all types of disabilities became visible in the community. I started to get help from people outside the disabled community. I started thinking of myself as a whole person. Attitudes changed in the community and life became easier for me. I was no longer seen as rebellious and non-conformist.

After I had been on the McLeod House Residents' Committee for about ten years, it became more powerful. We were getting information about how disabled people had helped themselves, where they got help and what different assistive aids were available. We told senior staff. I felt that I was a person on equal standing with anyone else. I had a lot to offer.

The committee at McLeod House seemed to be taken seriously

now. It became recognised by the matron and the administrative officer, and began to hold some power. We were asked what we thought the meals and snacks should be. You would think we would have already had a say in that, but no. At 'work', it was recognised that some of us weren't doing as well as our more physically abled counterparts. Some of us were put into a makeshift office. Positions were made for payroll clerks and secretaries. We were taught computer programming, commerce and tutoring skills.

Through being on this committee, I thought my placement at McLeod House was my destiny because I had found a role that gave me some satisfaction. But the committee also gave me ideas about what people with different handicaps were capable of doing. I learnt that people with disabilities a lot worse than mine were living in the community, playing sport and doing day-to-day tasks.

I never completely believed that my work on committees was helping people until things around the hostel started changing. Most of the changes were the result of decisions made by the committee, even if it was years later. Now all these improvements were happening, residents did not see a need for a committee any more. As there were no longer enough residents interested in forming a committee, a few of us joined with residents from Venee Burges House, the second hostel built by the Spastic Centre in the early seventies. All the residents were over twenty-one, and many of them over thirty-five. Although there seemed to be a large age gap between those at Venee Burgess and those at McLeod House, they still shared the same problems of living in an institution, so we had much in common.

I turned twenty-eight in 1986, the year of deinstitutionalisation. And so the deinstitutionalisation of McLeod House began. We started to be recognised as young adults who knew that there was a big wide world out there, and living in an institution and working in a sheltered workshop wasn't the norm. In 1987 I was invited to be on a steering committee. I was one of the two disabled representatives on it. There were now two hostels at the complex at Allambie Heights and twenty community houses in the nearby area. The North Shore was getting too expensive for the Spastic Centre to buy any more houses. The committee was looking at buying houses and setting up a workshop in the western suburbs. Being involved in all of this, I became determined to move into community housing, but my mother couldn't cope with the idea.

Meanwhile, I was visiting David at his new group house in Seaforth which he shared with two other young men. One of them was my ex-fiancé. That fact made an evening there very awkward. David moved to another house. This time he shared it with two young women. I felt more comfortable there. I knew David had no interest in either of them and that made evening meals more comfortable. I was spending more and more time with David. My parents went overseas a lot. I waited for them to go so I could spend more time at Seaforth.

16

Friday Nights

When my parents weren't overseas, my Friday night chore was coming home from work and making sure my dirty washing was folded correctly. I did this religiously every Friday afternoon to make the washing easier for my mother, even though she always found something I had folded incorrectly. Who folds their dirty washing anyway? I tried to rest between this mundane chore and being called into the bathroom, where I went obediently carrying my two towels and clothes for the evening. The bathroom was cluttered with wheelchairs and naked bodies, some of them in the bath or on the toilet, not caring about modesty. Although a soak in a hot bath was one of my favourite things of the day, I valued my privacy and almost dreaded bath time. After this ordeal, we started another chore: sitting in a circle in the lounge room facing a round dining room table covered in plates and food. We were clad in bibs and serviettes. After having an overcooked tea shovelled into our mouths, I raced to the front door where I waited for my mother or father to pick me up. I always anticipated their criticism in relation to my conversation. Spontaneous conversation was difficult after having spent a week living with people who could not verbally communicate.

My past attempts at asking my mother to move out into the community had failed miserably. I became cunning. I went home at weekends and told my family how well my friends were going in the outside world, in the hope they could see I was capable of doing the same thing. Being on residential committees helped me with assertiveness. I knew what I was talking about and stated so at various times over the weekend. I told them we were tapping into outside information centres, getting all kinds of information on how different disabled people helped themselves, where they went to get help and what assistive aids were available and that we gave senior staff this information to educate them. I became even more assertive, with help from rehabilitation officers. I was able to cut down my daytime resting to an hour a day and then attend more courses, such as self-assertiveness, being heard, how to develop listening skills, as well as having more time to tap into resources. Even with all this knowledge, it took me until I was twenty-nine to definitely decide to move out into a community house.

David moved to Armidale to start his first degree, in sociology and philosophy. I missed him. I still couldn't bring myself to tell my parents that I was definitely moving into the community and that I was in a committed relationship.

Meanwhile, my father and mother were overseas for a few months. In this time I agreed to move into a community house in the western suburbs of Sydney with two guys. The weekend my parents picked me up from the hostel after their trip away I told them I was moving. After an unpleasant weekend, I was taken back to the hostel with two suitcases of clothes and some of my personal belongings.

I lived in the group house in Winston Hills for eighteen months. This twenty-four-hour care home was an ordinary, mainstream Department of Housing house adapted for disabled people. Although it was staffed for twenty-four hours, there was a great emphasis placed on 'independence' – for instance, taking an hour to undress, shower and redress. I was used to spending a lot of time doing regular things. With my family I experienced a rich and fulfilling life as a child, with many activities. I didn't think it was the norm to spend four hours travelling to do six hours of menial tasks for under twenty dollars a week. I started to wonder about the emphasis on independence and what other people assumed was good for me. At the group house, we were taken to the local pub for an hour a week with our housemates, who I hadn't chosen to live with, let alone go out with. Though I was living in the community, so to speak, it wasn't really the ideal life.

17

Engagement and Marriage

David rang me from Armidale every Sunday afternoon. On a particularly cold afternoon when he rang, he asked me to marry him. I always wanted to marry, but to my surprise my answer was something like, 'Yeah, OK. Why don't we just live together?' It must have been the shock of him actually asking, even though I was kind of expecting something like that from him. We decided to get married six months later on 1 December 1990.

The engagement had to be made official and it is a moment that is still quite clear in my memory. David formally proposed at Kurrajong Lookout, halfway up to his parents' place at the top of the Blue Mountains. David produced a sock with a lump in the end. The lump was actually the engagement ring. David did not have the fine motor skills it took to pass me the box. Opening it was a challenge; somehow the ring box was taken out of the sock by one or both of us. We used the pile in the sheepskin seat cover of the David's car to help slide the ring on. I was engaged! The ring was an emerald set on a gold band with a diamond chip on either side.

The months between getting engaged and getting married were all go. There was the wedding dress and accessories, the engagement party and invitations and packing up my whole life in Sydney to arrange. David wanted to formally ask my parents for my hand in marriage as well, and we had wedding rehearsals and three trips to Armidale, all achieved in six months! All was eventually done. We ticked all the boxes and a few more. I will describe the preparations a little.

Two staff, Debbie and Tracey, from the Winston Hills group house decided to come up to help me on my big day. So that side of things was settled.

The invitations required some discussion. At first we only wanted to invite twelve people: our immediate families. Then parents suggested aunties and uncles, and we found when you invite one, it leads to fifty-four.

There were also many things that needed finishing up at the group home. The staff were wonderful in that respect. They also helped me get to the airport to fly to Armidale, took me to dress fittings and advised me on things to buy for my honeymoon and first night of marriage. My bridesmaid was a young woman, Helen, who had been working in the hostel's craft and recreation room. I kept in touch with Helen and she had taken me to her family home in Tamworth for her sister's engagement party. Helen was a great help with my wedding arrangements.

I needed to pick a dress of course. I believed in all or nothing and I wanted to be like my bride doll, Sharon, and wear a long white dress and veil. In hindsight, I should have picked a cool floral dress that was comfortable and could be worn again but I had high expectations of what a bride must look like. My bride doll, Sharon, had a beautiful white dress and veil. So I must too. I saved the money from my measly pension and got the works. It was a learning experience to say the least. I picked a beautiful dress but it was a size too small. The shop assistant said I needed to wear a corset. I immediately said yes, not thinking of the implications of the perspiration on a hot summer day. Then there were the trimmings. I didn't even think about those at first, things like headbands, veils, stockings, garters and shoes.

When I arrived in Armidale for the wedding, I lived in David's tiny flat for a few days. David moved into an old house just outside of Armidale. Then somehow the big day arrived.

On the day of the wedding, I had been awake since five a.m. staring at my beautiful dress and veil hanging on the dark wood stained, half-opened door. I got up and ate breakfast, showered and dressed in my underwear.

It was about nine a.m. when my father and sister came over. It was really no surprise to me that Michelle just appeared at our flat on the morning of the wedding having not formally accepted the invitation. We loved each other very much but for personal reasons had never been close. This wasn't a day for family problems, so they were all put aside. I had a spare bouquet so I made Michelle my second bridesmaid.

Then the phone rang. It was Mum. I could hear she was crying, but I ignored that. She talked about how she had sent me something old, something new, something borrowed and something blue, her pearls, a white lace handkerchief and a blue bird of happiness broach. (I permanently borrowed her white clutch bag.) And of course I had planned to wear them all. She wished me well and told me to enjoy my day.

After the phone call from my mother, I felt like my whole immediate small family was together. I felt calm and went on with my day. I had to marry Mr David Winston Heckendorf.

David's uncle drove Dad and Michelle and I up to St Mark's, the chapel at the University of New England. I directed them. It was up a hill near a white building. (There were many hills and white buildings.) We arrived ten minutes late. David was sitting at the back of the church as if sitting to attention. He wore a grey suit and black bow tie. My father pushed me down the aisle and David's best man, Peter, pushed him.

It was an intimate wedding. I was so nervous and excited, but I didn't cry.

Greg Burke was the chaplain who married us. He read from Corinthians 1:13:

> When I was a child, I spoke like a child, I reasoned like a child, I thought like a child; when I became a man, I gave up childish ways.

We wanted to have our photos taken under a big oak tree but

unfortunately everybody took our photo at the back of the chapel. Looking back on the photos now, David and I are amused. We forgot at the time that the disabled toilet was behind us and would be in the background of the photos. The oak tree would have been much better.

Our reception lunch was at the university restaurant. Andrew, who had been David's carer for about a year in Armidale, played in a bush band. They all offered to play at our reception for free, in their own time. Peter, David's friend from university, was his best man, and Helen was my bridesmaid.

Our wedding day ended up being like all the Christmases, birthdays and pool parties all rolled into one.

We were going out for dinner that evening but we were too tired and full. Lunch didn't finish until three p.m.! So that night David and I ordered takeaway to our country hotel room. Early the next morning we set off for Byron Bay and Wheel Resort, where we spent a week or so. Wheel Resort had a beautiful pool all set up to cater for the disabled and the pool was easy to get in and out of and we enjoyed swimming so much. We were accompanied by Andrew and his partner and their four-year-old son, Liam. This was the beginning of many years of happiness.

18

Rented Flat

In February 1993 David started a Law degree at the Australian National University (ANU). We spent two months at the old Gowrie Hostel, which is now called Fenner Hall, in Canberra. We were looked after by the Home Help Service. Administration staff and residents were helpful and caring, and always including us in meetings and activities. Although Fenner Hall was an institution, we really enjoyed the company and having the choice of joining in group activities or locking our door. Unfortunately, the living areas at Fenner Hall were too small to accommodate our needs. It was a strain on both us and our carers.

We made the unfortunate mistake of moving into shared accommodation – a group home with two other disabled people. As soon as we arrived we both thought the same thing – it was one very big step backwards, a step back from our home in Armidale to the group homes we had shared in Sydney. As a married couple living in this situation, it was made twice as bad by having experienced living in our own home. The choice to lock our door was taken away. I have always had carers and will always have them. I was mistaken to think all group homes were no longer run like mini-institutions. I am not against group housing or even small hostels but wherever people choose to live they should be cared for as individuals and their privacy should be respected.

I was able to depend on taxis to continue to enjoy shopping. Driving along the bike tracks, I had to keep looking over my shoulder, because the area was quite rough. But enjoying art, listening to talking books and spending time with David was often interrupted. We felt tied to this home with its hospital-like environment, always felt as if we were being watched, and usually we were. Even though I attended women's reading and writing classes at Woden TAFE, and also attended a writing workshop at Belconnen Library, we had to always come back to the house, where we were unable to be ourselves. It was a very stressful eight months.

We shared the house with one man who was missing half his insides and had to be tube-fed overnight. He was only in his fifties, but seemed as if he was approaching his eighties. The other guy was in his thirties, but had been institutionalised early in life, and went to a sheltered workshop for intellectually handicapped people. We had two quite large rooms to ourselves, one a study, and one a bedroom. Our tables and a small desk with our computers were in the study. Photos of David's graduation decorated the wall. It nearly felt like our old home. But the people in charge of the group houses hardly knew us. I'm sure there is a written description of a disabled person given out to administrators and their colleagues which is full of stereotypes and clichés. We weren't recognised as individuals. We wondered just who did care about the people in that house and houses like it.

Our hunt for alternative accommodation started the minute David came home from his last day of university. Most of our carers, support workers and close friends made dozens of phone calls and took us to look at an assortment of flats. It wasn't until the Monday before Christmas that we found our flat in Lyons on the south side of Canberra. We were in the dark dingy flat by lunchtime. It was all ours and we loved it, despite the dusty psychedelic carpet and tiny rooms. It was similar to the first flat we had in Armidale. Friends helped us move in the following morning and left it in chaos. But we didn't mind. We were so relieved to be out of the group house.

19

Life in Canberra

It turned out to be a very creative place and time in our lives. I got the opportunity through Belconnen Library and Mary Hutchinson to publish a few of my short stories in a local community book, *Caring Words*. Then I got the opportunity to publish some of my cartoons in *My guide to the individual support package* by Keris Delaney.

This led to me enrolling in a drawing course, and then a diploma in Visual Art at ANU. My main body of work involved nude self-portraits. I let some of them blur, to show my movements, using longer exposures. My aim was to show that people with disabilities could be sexual beings just like any other person. I also made computer-generated work taken by scanning photographs and manipulating them with filters. I did a series on my interpretation of evolution. I made a montage with images of the sort of movement I had in water, and played with the irony of the restrictions my callipers gave me when I was more able. I also had a camera stand fitted to my wheelchair. I shot a series called 'Beauty and Barriers' on the irony of the beauty of nature versus the barriers it creates. I used to drive my chair from Curtin to Acton and had some hair- raising experiences: for instance, you can't get away from a snake if Lake Burley Griffin is on one side and a steep embankment is on the other.

In the meantime, David worked as a policy officer on the other side of Canberra. Though I was busy making a lot of artwork, it was my daily ritual to ring David after lunch, even if he only had time to say a quick hello. I rested every day after lunch and still do. When you are sitting in a wheelchair all day, it's good for your body to have a break out of it. So I would lie down and listen to the local radio station. This also relaxed me. I needed to do this to help manage my energy levels. And some days I had lunch with David at a restaurant near where he worked.

In the May of 2007, we moved into our town house in Lyons in the central south of Canberra. David was still working in the north side of Canberra when we moved. We were offered the Lyons town house when David was in hospital for three months, recovering from a hip operation. I was still giving the occasional talk at disability-related events, but managed to visit David every day, bar two, in hospital. It was convenient moving to Lyons because it was a quick wheelchair ride to the local shopping centre. It was handy not just for shops but for banks and other facilities. We liked our cup of coffee at the local café too, and we felt that it educated the staff who served us there, as although we have particular needs, we are just like any other couple. The staff got used to it. They served us and other people in minority groups, such as the elderly, and we helped the staff learn patience and understanding of people in different situations.

The best part of the first year in our new home was spent researching a holiday in Hawaii. With special needs to consider, you don't just book a hotel room and a plane seat. You have to look into accessible transport and accommodation. Little things like where to hire a wheelchair charger and where to get compatible power point adapters had to be done. We managed it all and had a wonderful trip. The highlight for me was having a swim in the Pacific Ocean in a wheelchair designed for the water. Although it was a fairly rough swim and an accidental mouthful of salty water was horrible, I had achieved my ambition of having a swim off the islands of Hawaii.

David moved to the Department of Health. It was only five minutes away. I could join him for lunch and sometimes morning tea. This made me feel more secure. Rather than being on the other side of Canberra, he was only a few minutes away. I could go and see him if I had a big problem, but I had to be very careful to respect his work environment.

I signed up to Facebook in 2008. A friend asked me by email to join so that I could follow her overseas trip. I now have over a hundred 'friends', many of whom I don't even know, and I'm sure many people can identify with this. As neither David or I can physically play a board game, we use Facebook to do so. We also interact with family and friends. But this doesn't consume our day. Nothing replaces face-to-face interactions and human touch.

20

Broken Foot

A month before my fiftieth birthday, I slipped and fell down, sitting on my left foot and breaking it in three places. Even though I heard bones crunch, the ambulance officers didn't want to take me to hospital, but I insisted. I had been getting out of bed to go to the bathroom. I had stood up but not clearly seen the horizontal bar from the vertical rail that was bolted from floor to ceiling about three feet away from my bed. I was starting to fall on a regular basis so the ambulance officers knew me. They didn't want to take me to hospital but I think when I said I had heard a crunch they believed me. Eleven days later, I was discharged from hospital with a sling, hoist and commode chair. It wasn't the injury that kept me in hospital, it was the organisation of the extra care I needed.

For the next six months, the sole of my foot was bruised. Community physiotherapists tried to get me wearing shoes and to bear weight. Though I wanted my independence back, I believe this hurt my foot more. My GP sent me to a sports doctor, who ordered me a few more scans, located the bruising and had me in hospital to reset broken bones. I believe the bones had been pressing on nerves, and to this day I have swelling and nerve pain.

After the operation on my left foot, I concentrated on taking the Canberra Hospital to the Discrimination Office. I wanted to sue the hospital for negligence. I believed that if they had done my MRI when I was in hospital my foot would have healed more quickly and I might even be able to weight bear today. An independent assessment was done by Sydney University and a doctor who specialised in cerebral palsy wrote a report saying I probably missed the pole due to my shaking arms. I received an apology letter from the CEO of the Canberra Hospital saying they were sorry for the inconvenience or something to that effect. I could have pursued this more but one person can't fight Canberra Hospital, and I had to get on with life.

I can't transfer into or out of my wheelchair any more and rely heavily on carers. I guess it almost goes without saying that our care hours have increased. Our days are highly organised.

I have high physical dependencies. Interviewing carers is a daunting task for all involved. With the assistance of a coordinator from the company we got our care from, we now interview and employ our personal care staff. We realise this can be an unfamiliar situation for potential carers. More often than not, fear of the unknown creeps into the situation of meeting someone for the first time. We think this is especially so for someone who is unfamiliar with our jerky movements and slurred speech.

Our disabilities have increased and so has our support, mine more than David's. It happens with most cases of cerebral palsy, but I must not dwell on it and keep doing whatever I can, while I can.

21

Intimacy

In the first fifteen years of our marriage, David and I had a very intimate and active personal life in the bedroom. Because of the wear and tear cerebral palsy puts on your body, we both had hip replacements. Intimacy became more difficult. We took the plunge and hired a sex worker to assist us with our personal life in the bedroom. The decision to have a third person in the bedroom wasn't an easy one. It took us a long time to get used to it. It is still a controversial part of our life and remains a topic of heated conversation with many people.

22

Activities Today

I go to gym twice a week. The gym is run by the Cerebral Palsy Alliance and is specially fitted out so wheelchairs can get to the machines. Seats are fully adjustable and can be taken away for those in a wheelchair, and then locked back in for more able clients.

I usually attend a class on Australian history at the University of the Third Age, commonly known as U3A. It is a group of intelligent people over the age of fifty. Many of us have university degrees and speak each week. We have morning tea and chat.

I have always taken pride in doing the grocery shopping. These days, I am actually getting a bit tired of it, although I think it is important for me to know how the house is run, and it is as important as physical exercise and socialising. It is my way of taking responsibility for our well-being and taking care of David, and also just taking care of both of our health.

23

Canberra Now

Back through the vortex to our overgrown Japanese maple which covers my climbing rosebush now. We have been in our Canberra town house for the best part of eleven years. We are still sitting in our office at the same window. But we are now off on our next adventure. We are soon to begin the next part of our lives. We are almost up to the point of packing up my delicate ornaments and moving to Brisbane to be closer to family and friends. We have researched land and houses, designed our own home and we are ready to move to a new city in a new state.

Appendix

As I grew older, the importance of McLeod House became clearer to me. Funds to children with disabilities were being cut. I could only think of how lucky I had been having the beginning I did with the Spastic Centre. I was asked by the University of the Third Age to give a presentation. So I talked about how the Spastic Centre came to be.

A brief history of the Spastic Centre of NSW

(Research for this talk was completed in The National Library, Cerebral Palsy Alliance Website and through social networks.)

I will be using the word 'spastic' a lot today. It is a word we are all probably used to hearing in the school yard used as a nasty word. Spastic is actually a type of cerebral palsy. There are five different types of cerebral palsy. I am an athetoid. I have also developed dystonia. When the word spastic is used colloquially, it usually just means some kind of cerebral palsy. Spasticity is found in stroke patients too. Its characteristics are stiffness or rigidity.

You can't begin to understand the history of the Spastic Centre of NSW without knowing Neil and Audrie McLeod. If it wasn't for the birth of their first daughter, Jenny, there would be no Spastic Centre as we know it today. Jennifer was born in Perth in the 1930s. Mr McLeod was at the war when Jennifer was born. Mrs McLeod was told by paediatricians to forget about her daughter, Jenny, put her in a home and forget about her. Mrs McLeod fought them to take Jenny home, holding her floppy head while she took hours to feed, and exercising her stiff limbs. I remember hearing people being told this when I was young: to put your child in an institution and forget them. Until the 1970s, this was just a part of everyday life. It didn't upset me. I think there is a place for well-run institutions.

Mrs McLeod encouraged Jenny to listen to the ABC radio musical show for children. She got Jenny to join in, playing simple musical instruments as best she could. A journalist from Perth's ABC radio asked Mrs McLeod for an interview about Jenny's life at home. She consented, and it resulted in perhaps one of the first verified findings that children with cerebral palsy could participate in a mainstream activity, even though they needed very specialised care in other areas.

Music became recognised as an important part of the lives of children with cerebral palsy. I remember listening to the ABC radio once a week in primary school. Once a term we were taken into the Town Hall to what I thought was a horrible orchestral concert. I wished I paid more attention back then.

A neurologist, Dr Carlson, who had cerebral palsy himself, came out from the USA to visit New Zealand and Australia, and share his knowledge of institutions for children with cerebral palsy. This included everything from education to hydrotherapy. He was influential in Australian people's understanding of how to treat and educate children with cerebral palsy.

In his travels back from the war, Mr McLeod came across a motorised wheelchair and while in Kalgoorlie he came across a child's pedal car, the sort which was still used for exercise when I was at school. I am unsure of the order but also on his travels Mr McLeod met Mr Arthur Sullivan in New York. He was a well-dressed travel merchant who offered Mr McLeod a property in Mosman, Sydney. This seems like an extraordinary story. From memory, the building started in 1946. Fathers of around forty children helped build the school.

It is documented that the first 'button day' was in 1946. They then sold for two, one and sixpence. I remember the mothers being ferried into town with cardboard trays around their necks, like they had in the picture theatres. They travelled into the heart of Sydney to sell buttons. These buttons were in a ribbon-like shape. Various colours represented various prices. I could never figure out why it was called button day when they were selling pieces of paper.

There are slightly contradictory accounts of the location of the first school. Mr McLeod's book *Nothing is impossible* states it was in Queen Street, Mosman, but Spastic Centre lore suggests the first school building was in Glover Street and was up and running in 1946. At the Spastic Centre, the children slept in splints to help stretch their muscles. The use of braces, plasters and splints was used to try and assist tiny children to walk.

Children with cerebral palsy could have one limb affected or their whole body. Sixty years ago, children with cerebral palsy weren't expected to live to become adults. Schools and hostels were rare. Although they seemed cruel, they were a lot better than the large warehouse-like institutions or lying around in your family's back room. So, contrary to many individuals' belief, the children who were at these schools were the lucky ones. We travelled each day to Mosman in an old army bus from different parts of Sydney. Each week, most of us had travelled the equivalent to a trip across Australia.

The first Miss Australia Quest was in 1954. It supported the Spastic Centre. It ran until the late 80s or 90s. Then it was seen as being sexist, and a glorified meat market. Men were allowed to join the Quest until the early 2000s. Then it was banned.

As mentioned in *Through the Years*, the Hostel for Country Children of NSW was opened in 1957 The same year, Centre Industries opened. There, able-bodied adults worked alongside the less abled, in a factory-like setting.

Five years later, parents formed a board of directors. My father was a member of it for over twenty years. McLeod House was built to be a boarding school-like facility for around sixty children with cerebral palsy and parents of babies with CP, plus a primary school and a few beds for adults. There were as many adults as there were children. The school had to be closed to make room for the increasing number of adults. The children were being bussed over to the also bulging at the seams school at Mosman. When the hostel was built, it was not thought that we were to grow up into quite healthy adults.

A second school was built at Allambie Heights in the 70s. There was much rivalry between the two schools. They were both the best. Because David did most of his schooling at Allambie, we have many healthy debates on this subject. A second school and hostel was opened in 1974. This hostel accommodated around fifty adults.

In 1983, the Stewart Centre was opened at Chowder Bay, Newcastle. To my knowledge, it was a school and treatment centre. I am unsure what it is now. A year later, Mr McLeod received an OBE. His wife had received one the year before.

The Marconi Centre was built in western Sydney. It ran twenty-two group homes for independent living. This is recorded as having happened in 1995, but I lived in a group home in western Sydney in 1989, the year before David and I got married.

Without the birth in 1930 of Jenny to her devoted parents, Mr Neil and Mrs Audrie McLeod, people with cerebral palsy might still be living in warehouse-like institutions. These do exist in some Slavic and Russian countries today. Not only did the McLeods start the Spastic Centre in Sydney, they had very close relationships with Japan and probably other countries I am unaware of, so their contribution and influence was international. With the Spastic Centre, now known as the Cerebral Palsy Alliance, in a bright new building overshadowing the run down McLeod House, there are many changes. New young therapists and departments fill the shiny new glass and steel buildings. Unfortunately, McLeod House lies in its shadows, with its future being debated. (This was the case in 2012 when I gave this talk. Since then, McLeod House has become an aged care facility.)

Lightning Source UK Ltd.
Milton Keynes UK
UKHW041227270120
357678UK00002B/524